W9-BDV-386

EMBRACE

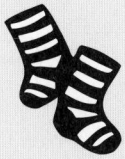

This Journal Belongs To:

EMBRACE

A Pregnancy Journal

Nikki McClure

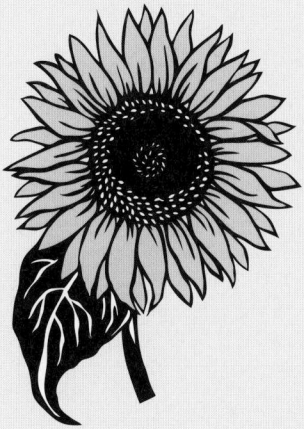

SASQUATCH BOOKS
SEATTLE

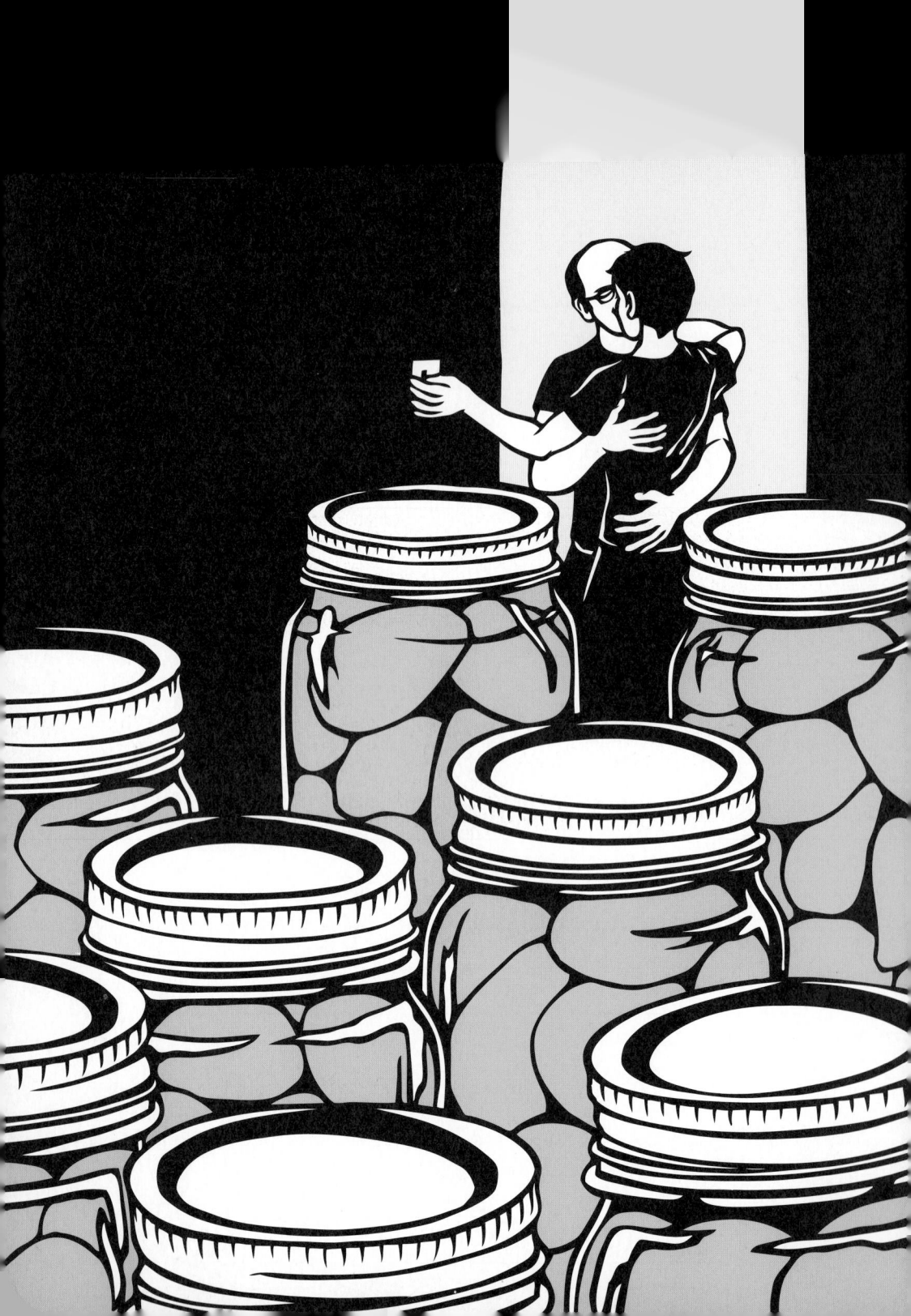

DESIRE

how I wanted a baby

the yearning

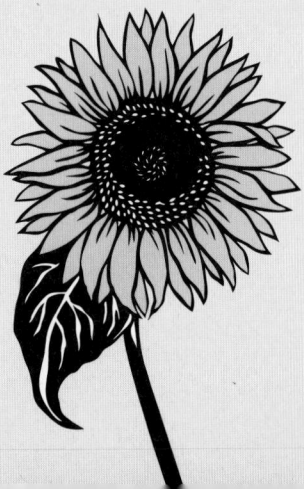

the searching

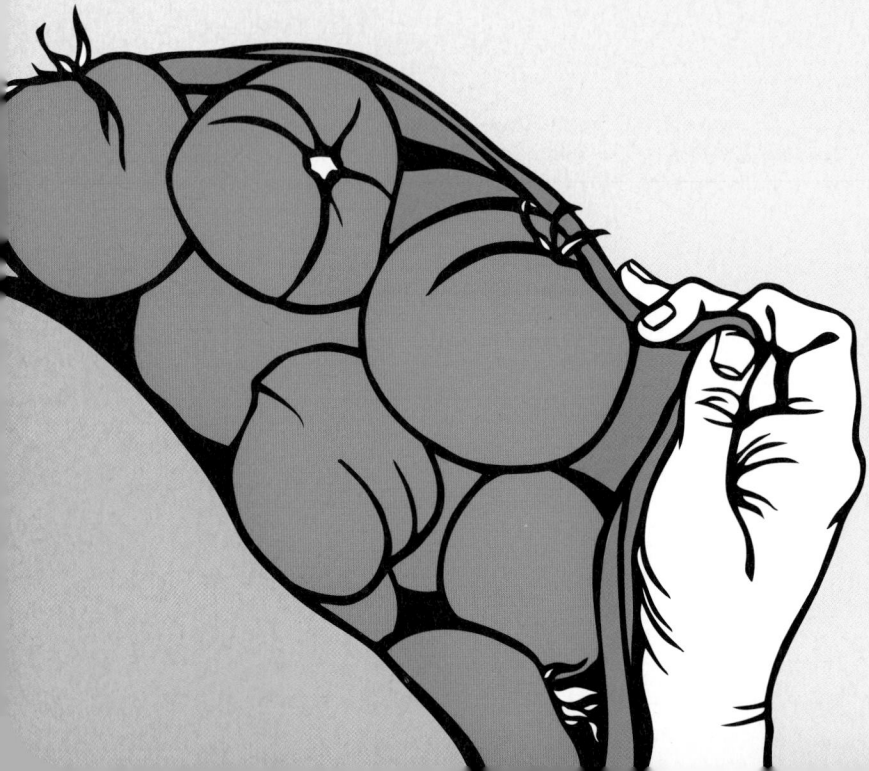

DISCOVER

how I knew I was pregnant

early inklings of this baby inside

telling my partner

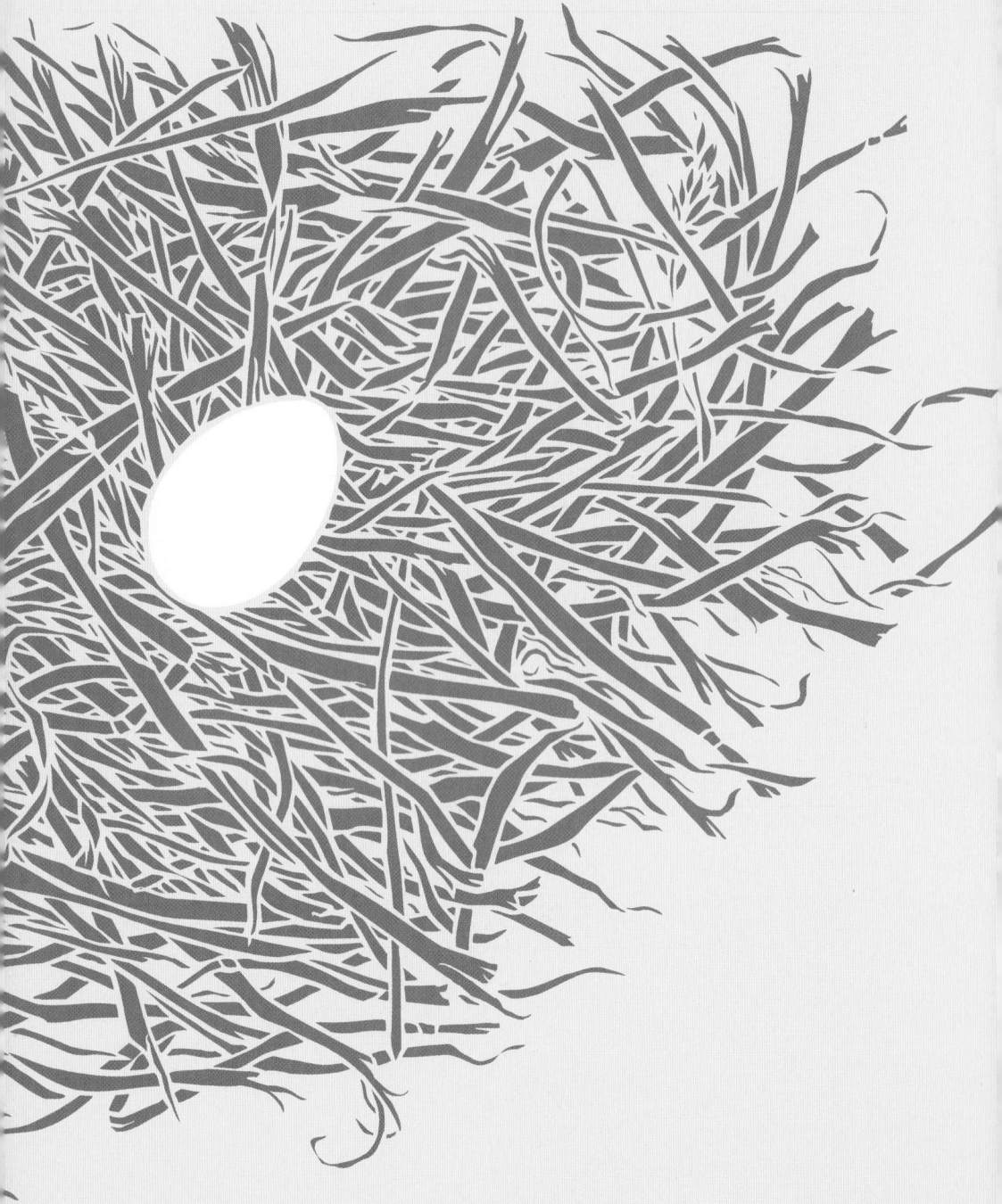

EMBRACE

preparing for this new adventure

excitement, worry, joy, fear

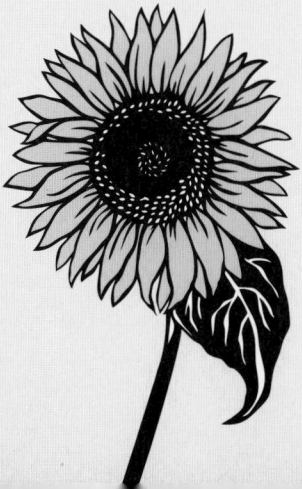

laughing, thinking, embracing

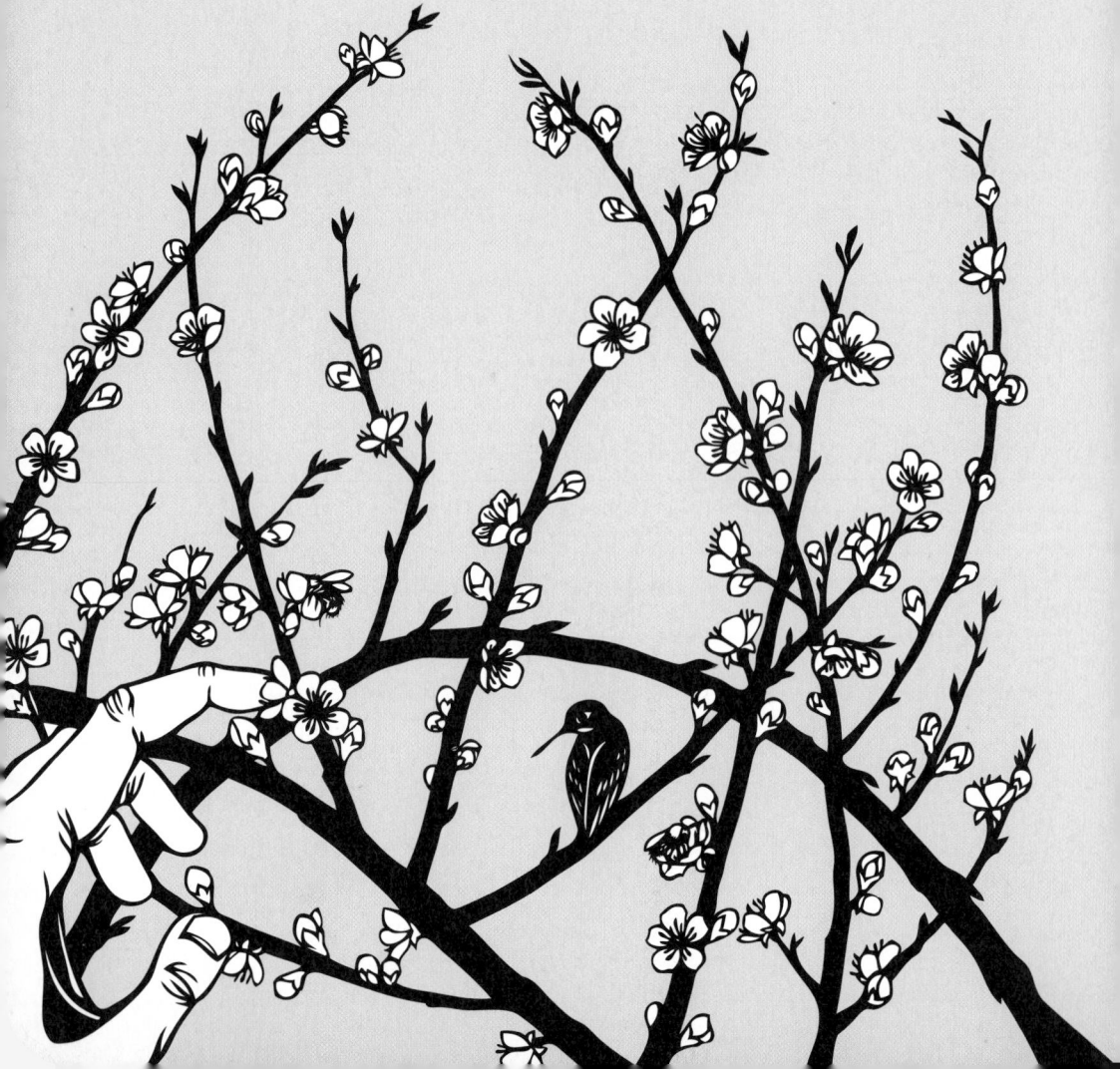

GROW

it is all I can think of

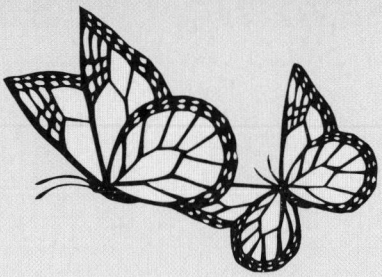

I am pregnant. I am pregnant. I am pregnant.

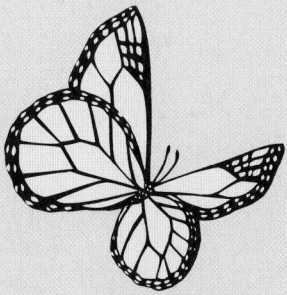

My breasts are so big!

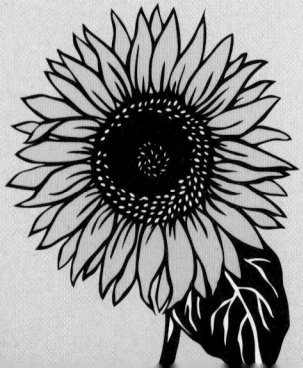

Who have I told this secret to?

I am pregnant!!!!!

special places to rest at home and work

take a walk with my best friend

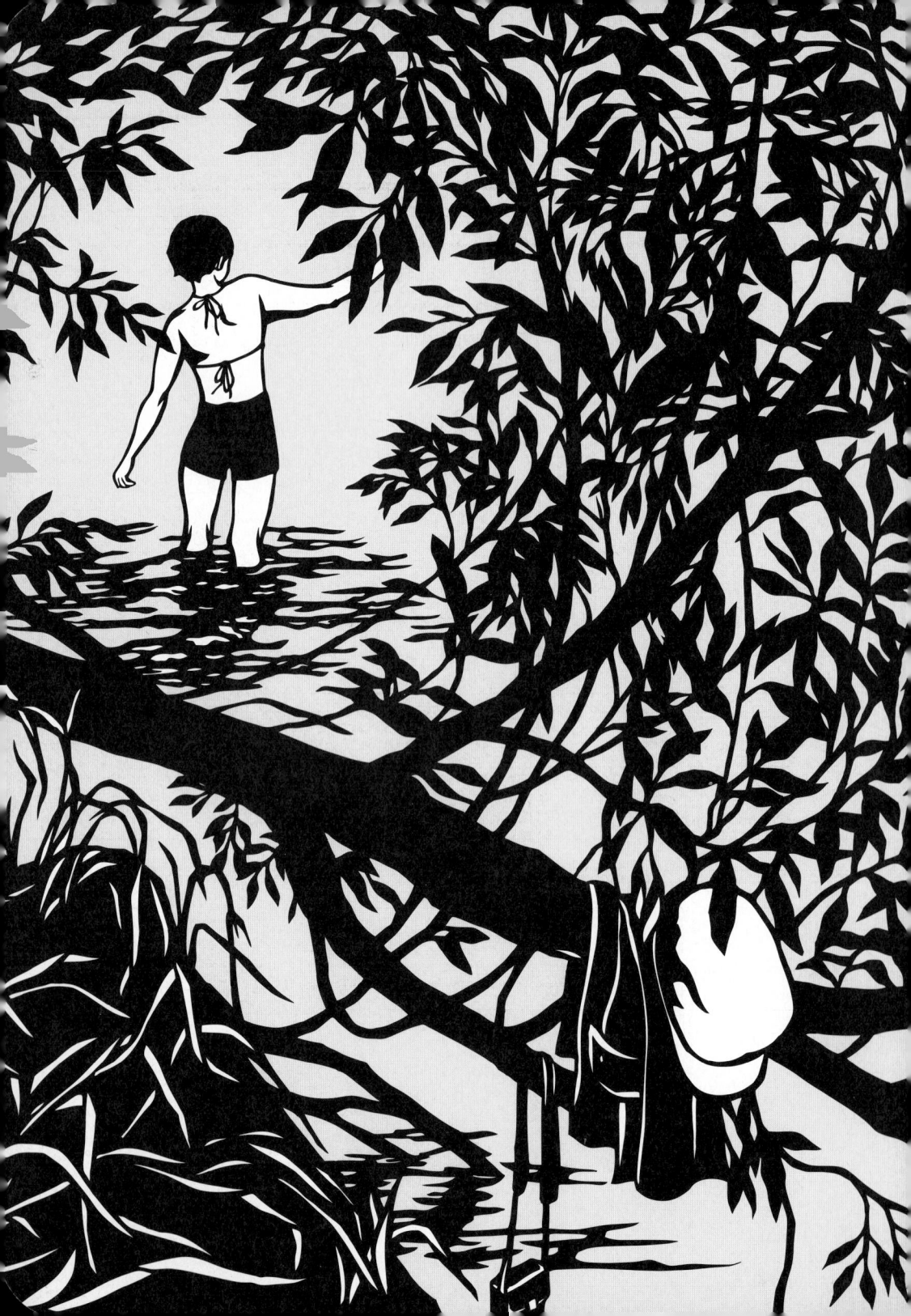

sharing my body is work

2nd MONTH

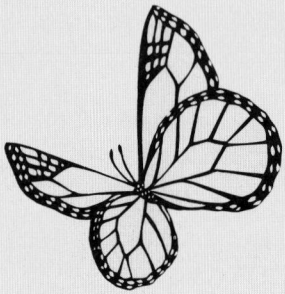

what I crave

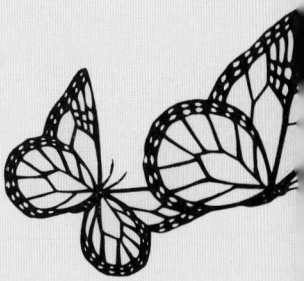

things that make me queasy

taking care of myself

searching for a midwife or doctor

good food to grow a strong baby

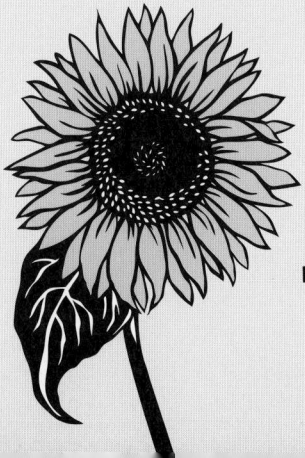

my baby's heart is beating now

Am I showing?

how tired I am

love the love

shouting it out to the world

sharing the news

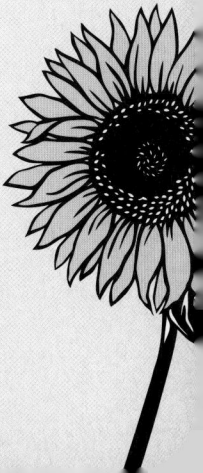

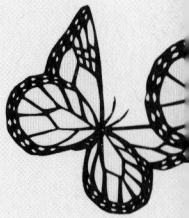

celebrating this new life inside me

accepting and growing

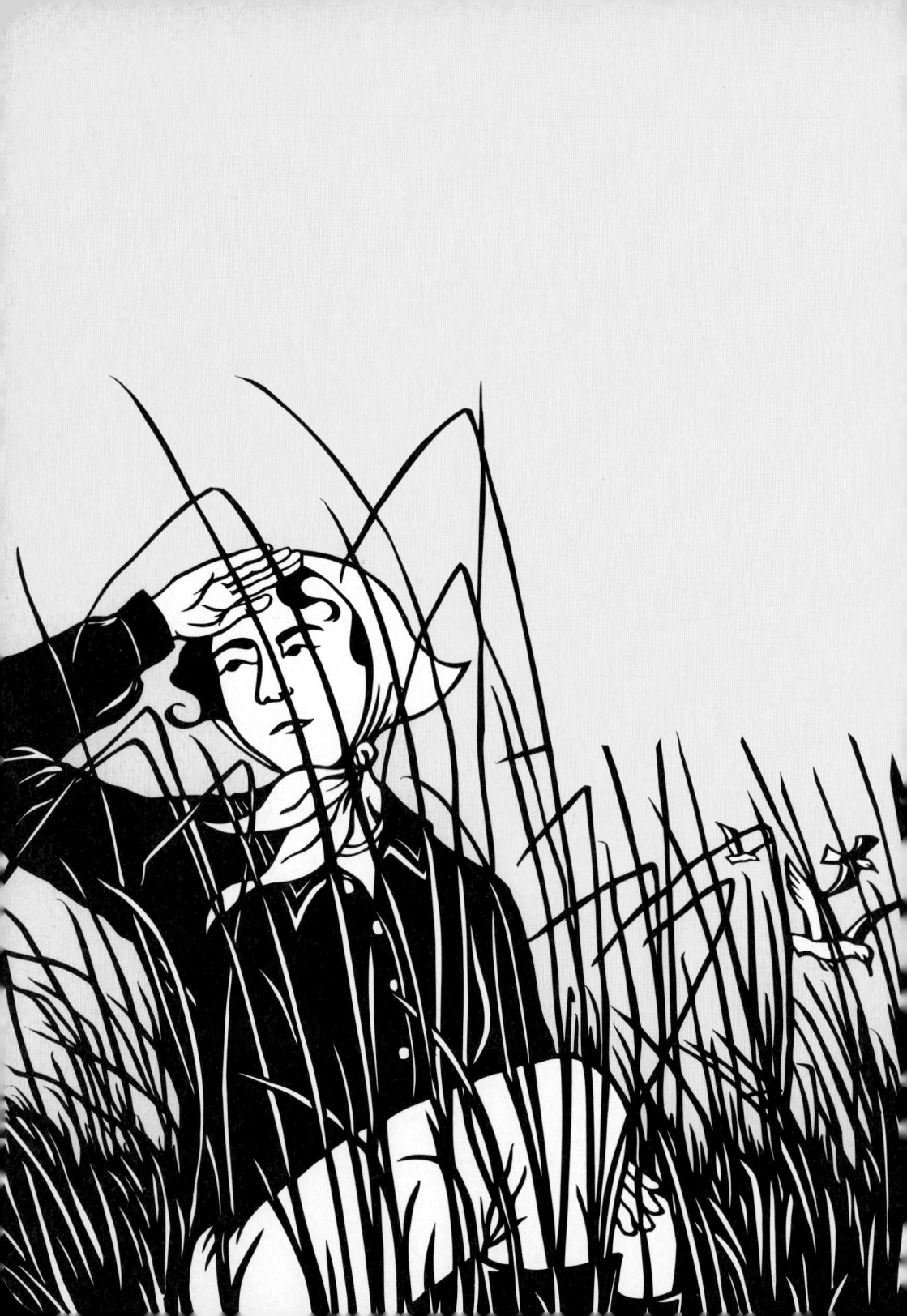

this is really happening

my energy returns, yoga, walk, swim

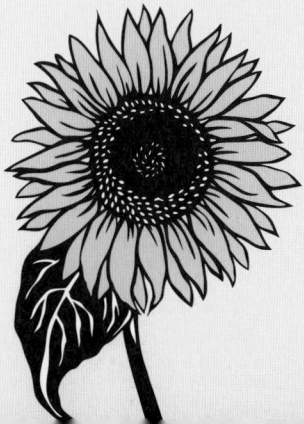

glow, love, smile all day

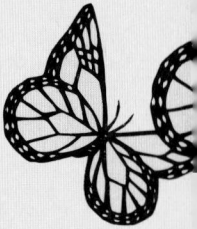

my belly cannot be contained

rubber bands hold my pants on
for one more week

feeling my baby fluttering inside

deepening connection to my partner
and support from my community

feelings about my family

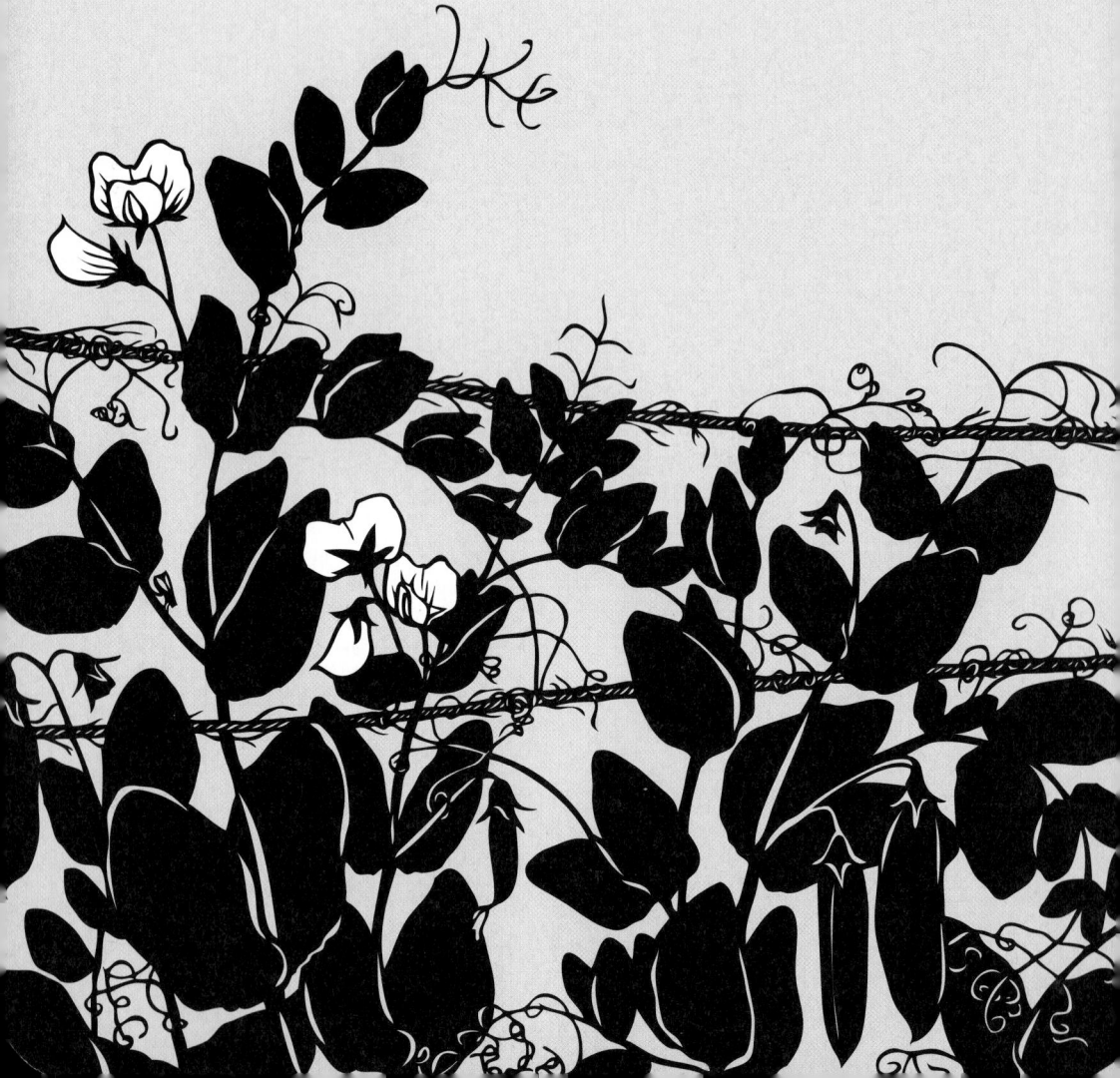

5th MONTH
gravity is shifting

I can see you.

ultrasound images

your nose, fingers, feet

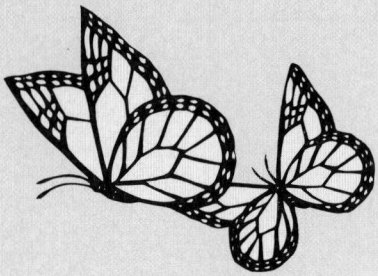

new aches and cramps

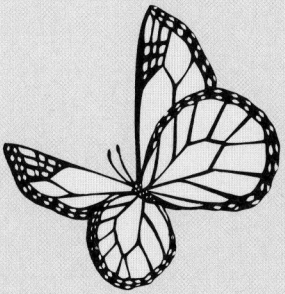

foot rubs, friends, naps, more food

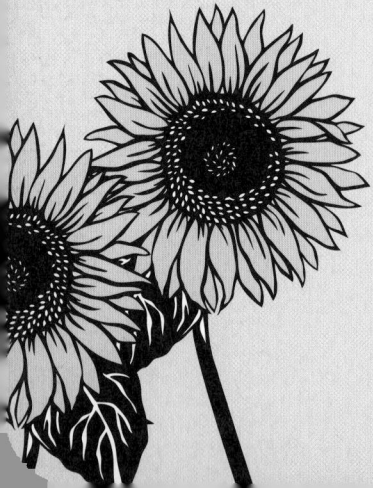

my favorite snacks

I am confident and beautiful.

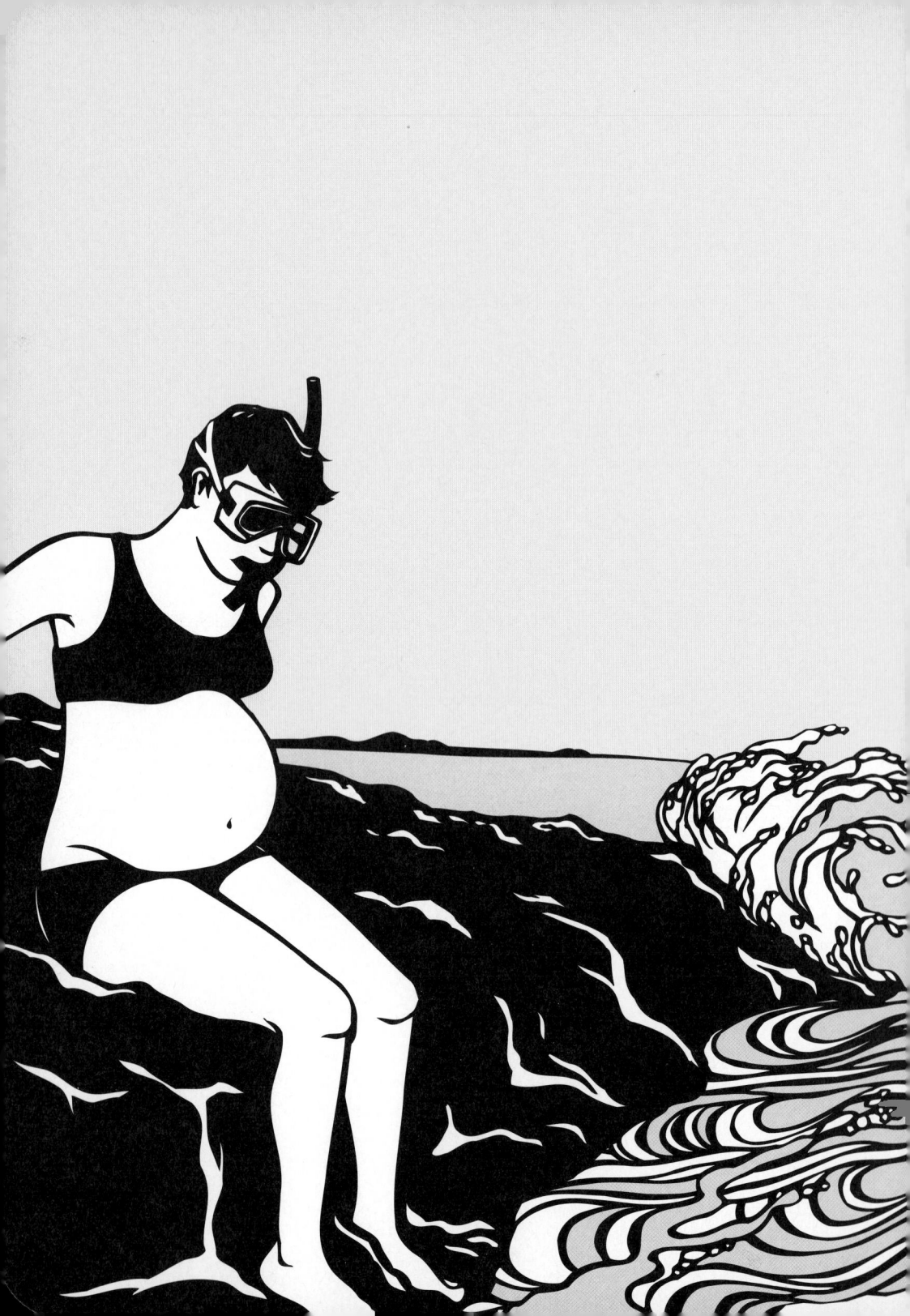

What kind of mother will I be?

What was my mother like?

What was I like as a baby?

my pillow arrangement

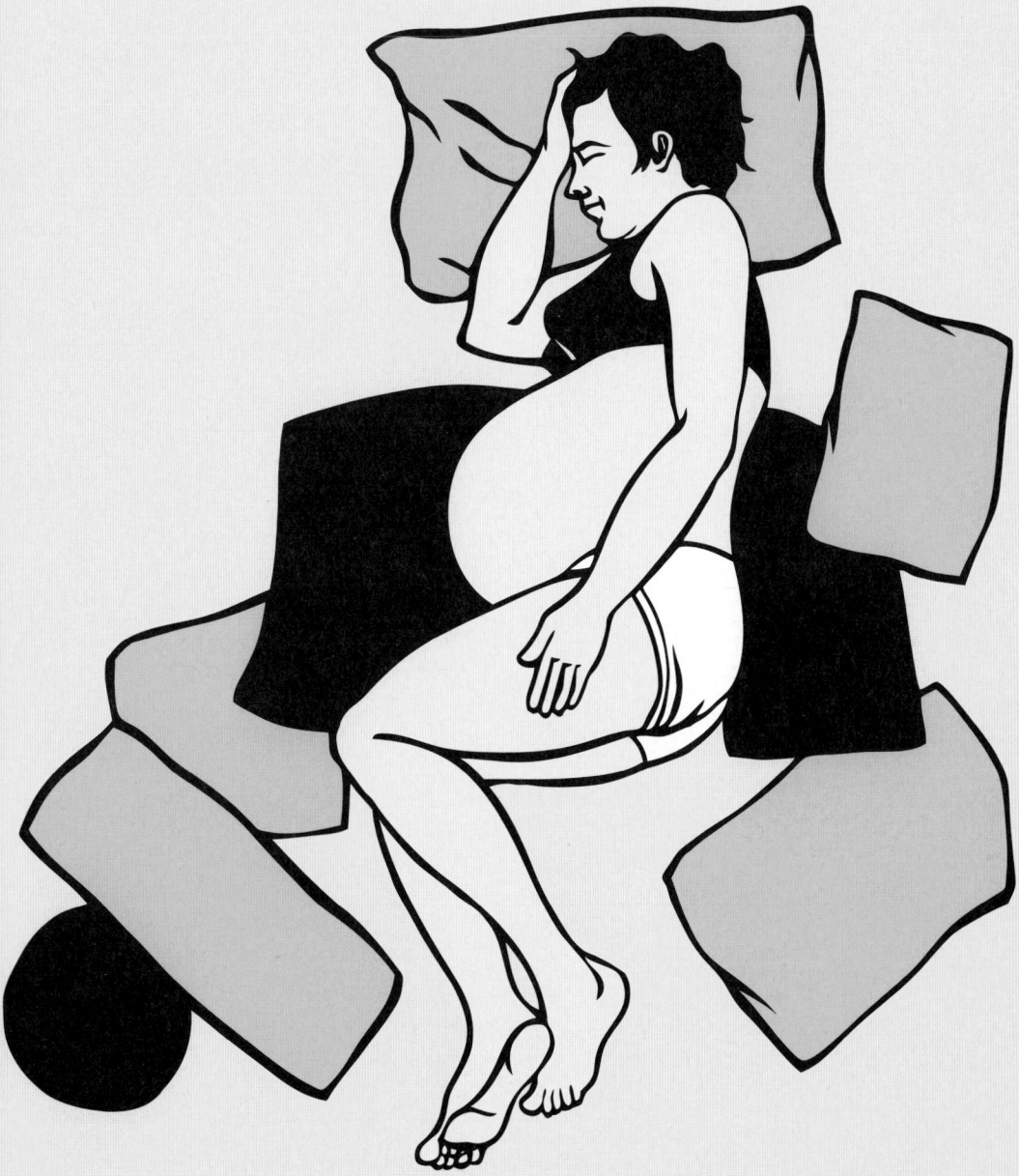

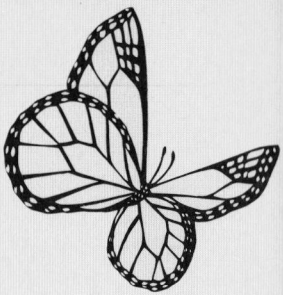

One last getaway trip?

a babymoon

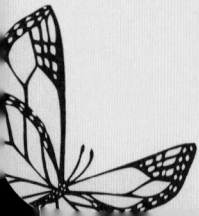

grow, grow, grow, and drink nettle tea

crumble dried nettles and mint leaves into teapot,
add hot water,
steep for five minutes,
pour and add honey

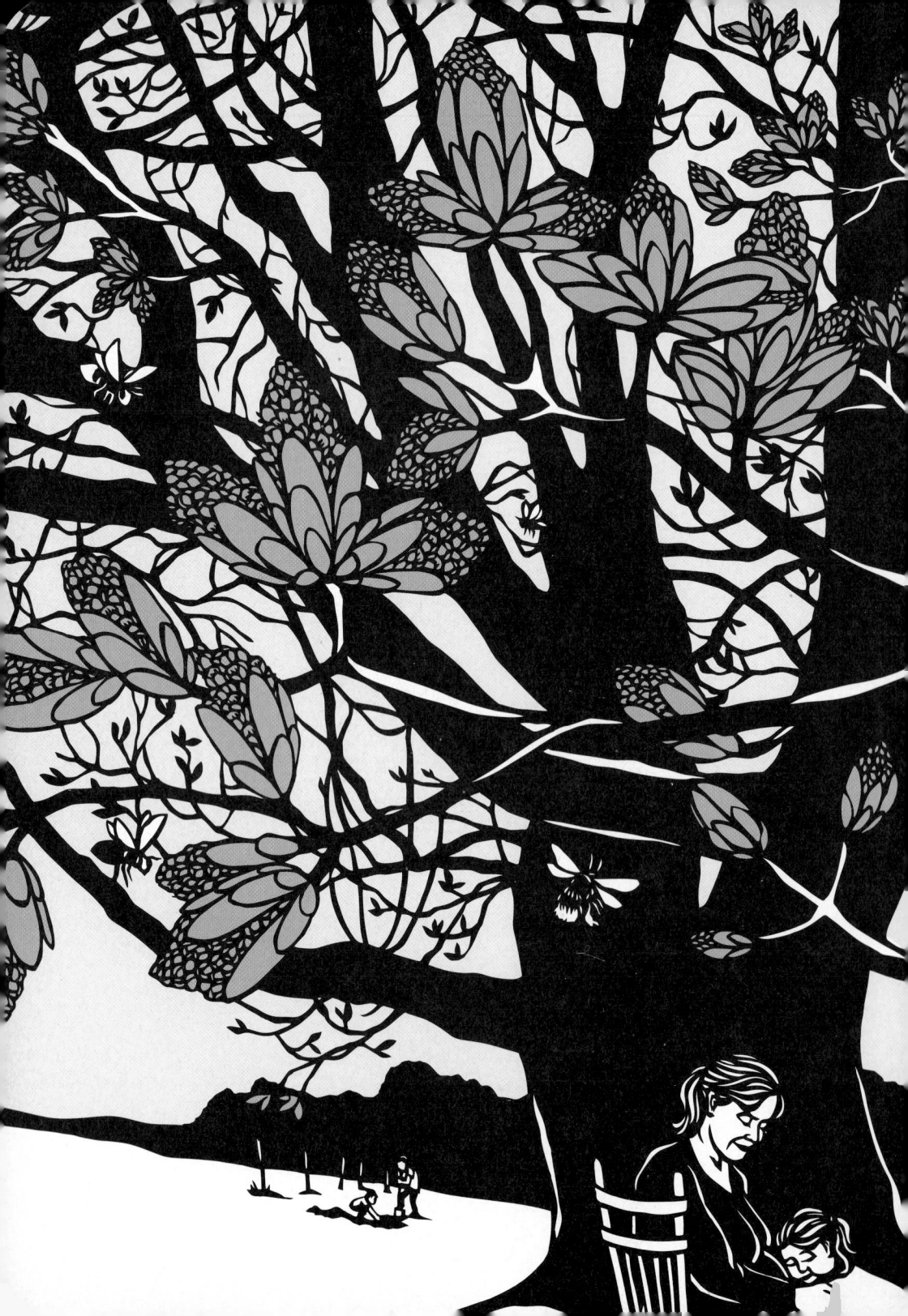

7th MONTH

Get things done!

Diaper service? Freeze a lasagna?

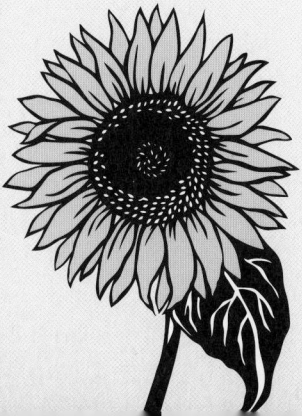

Birth class? Massage?

talk to other mothers

especially my own

see a movie

make a movie

go for a long walk and take a long nap

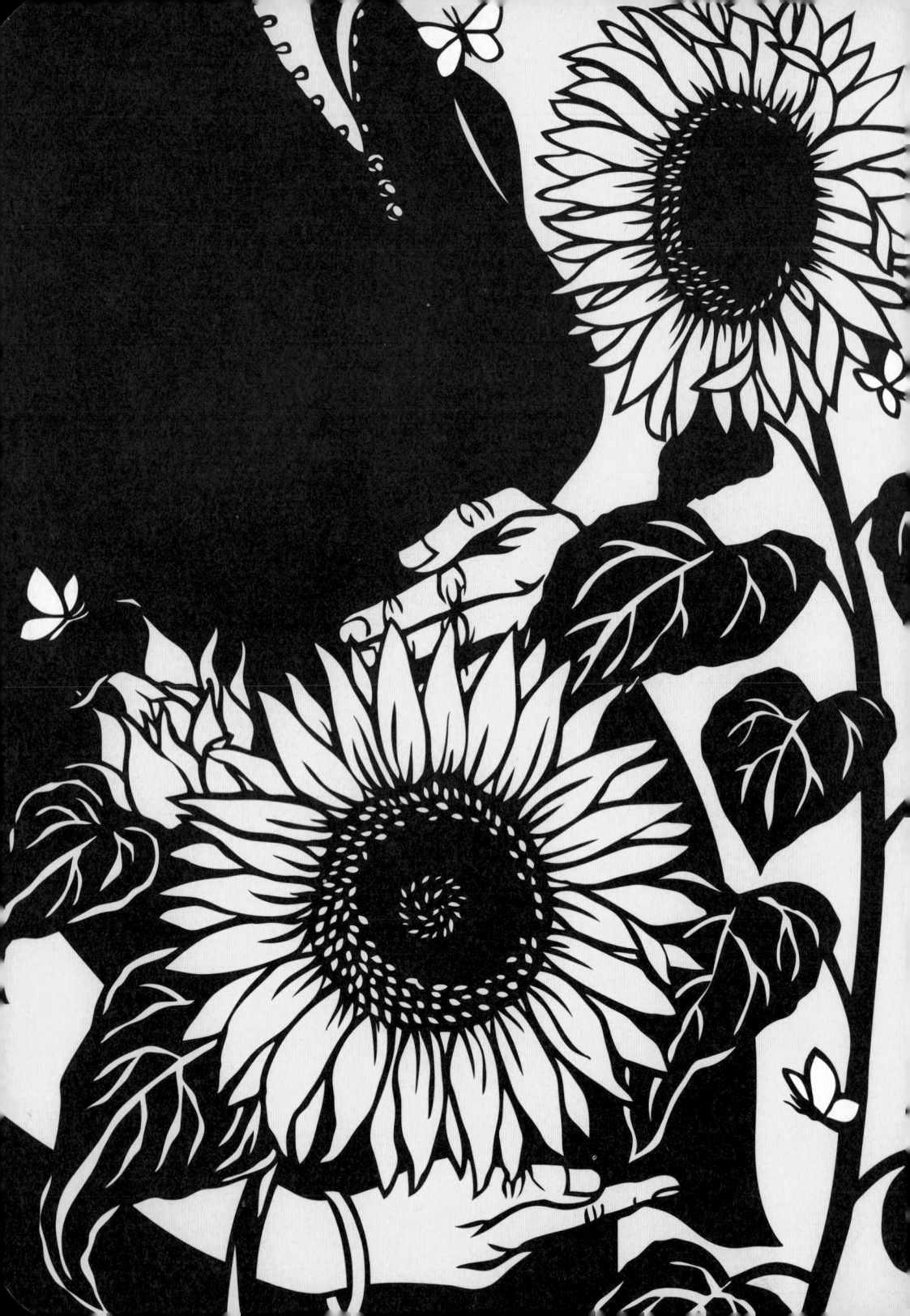

I am so pregnant.

baby shower plans

and all those good wishes

Who has felt the baby move? Hiccup?

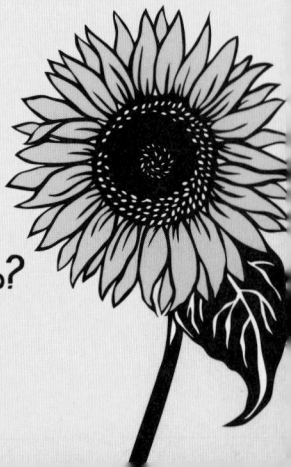

searching for my baby's doctor

ADVICE FROM FRIENDS

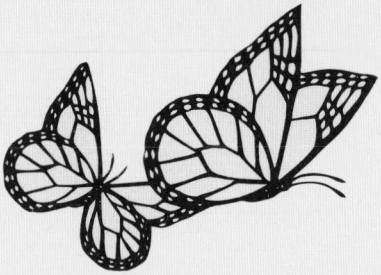

return library books

get a car seat ready

for every day past your due date,
do something nice for yourself

ADVICE FROM STRANGERS

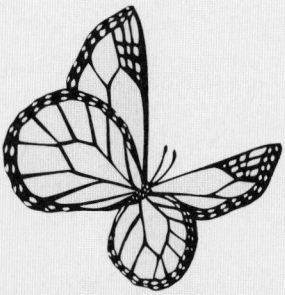

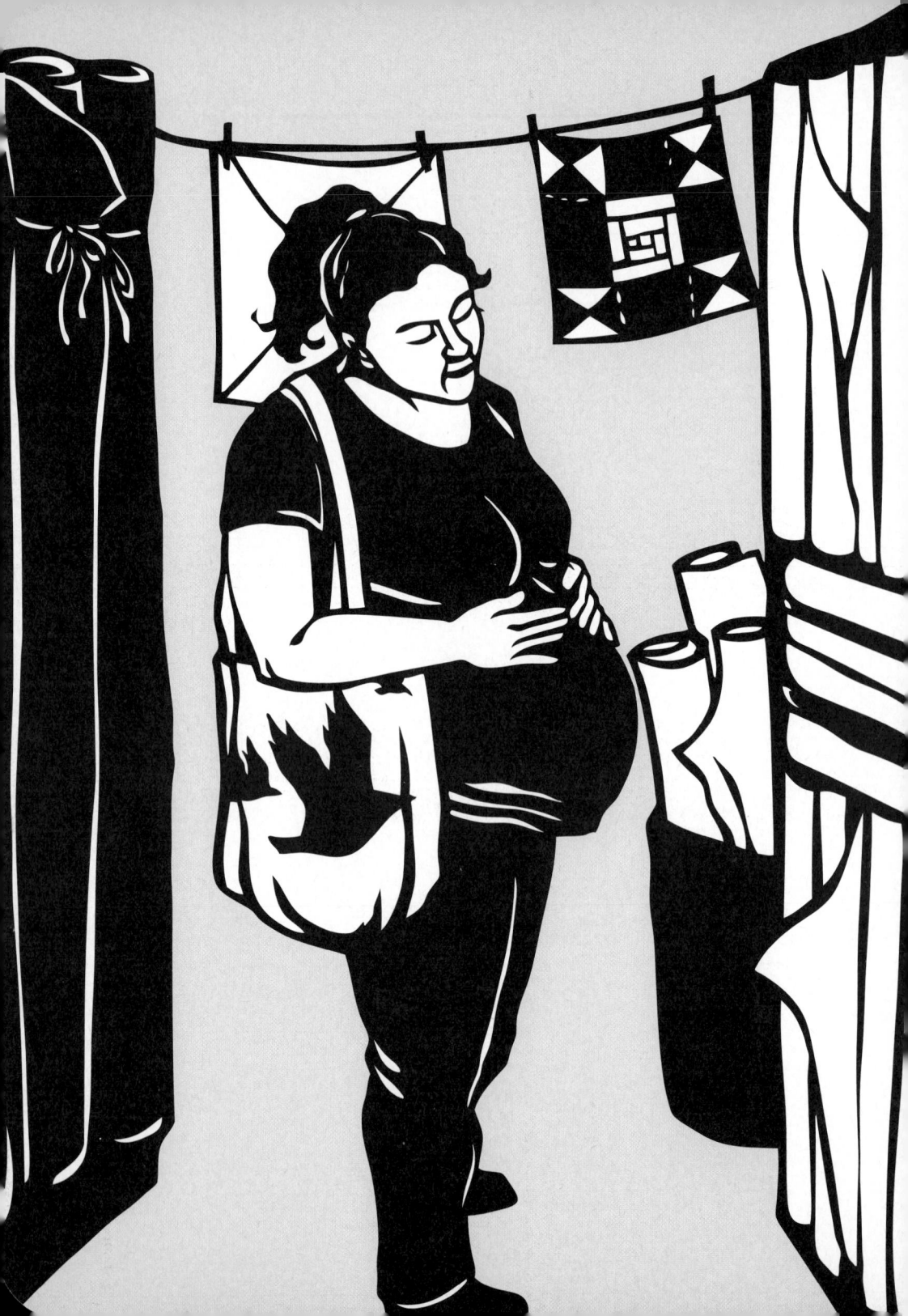

9th MONTH
waiting

my birth plan

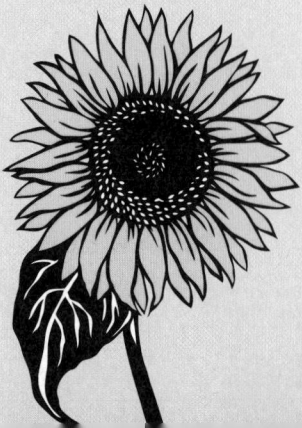

nesting, preparing the burrow

drawing of my belly button

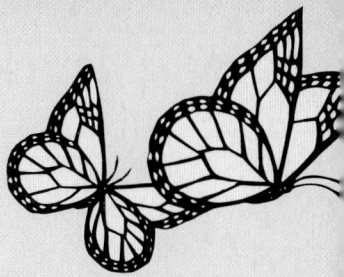

drawing of baby ready inside

WAYS TO PASS THE TIME

start a quilt that will never be finished

rest!

climb a mountain

clean out the refrigerator

talk to friends for hours

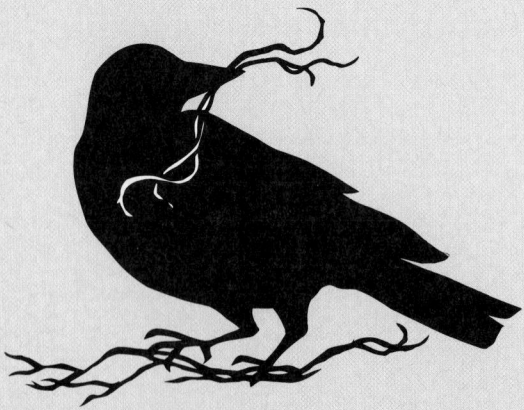

the summoning, the call to begin

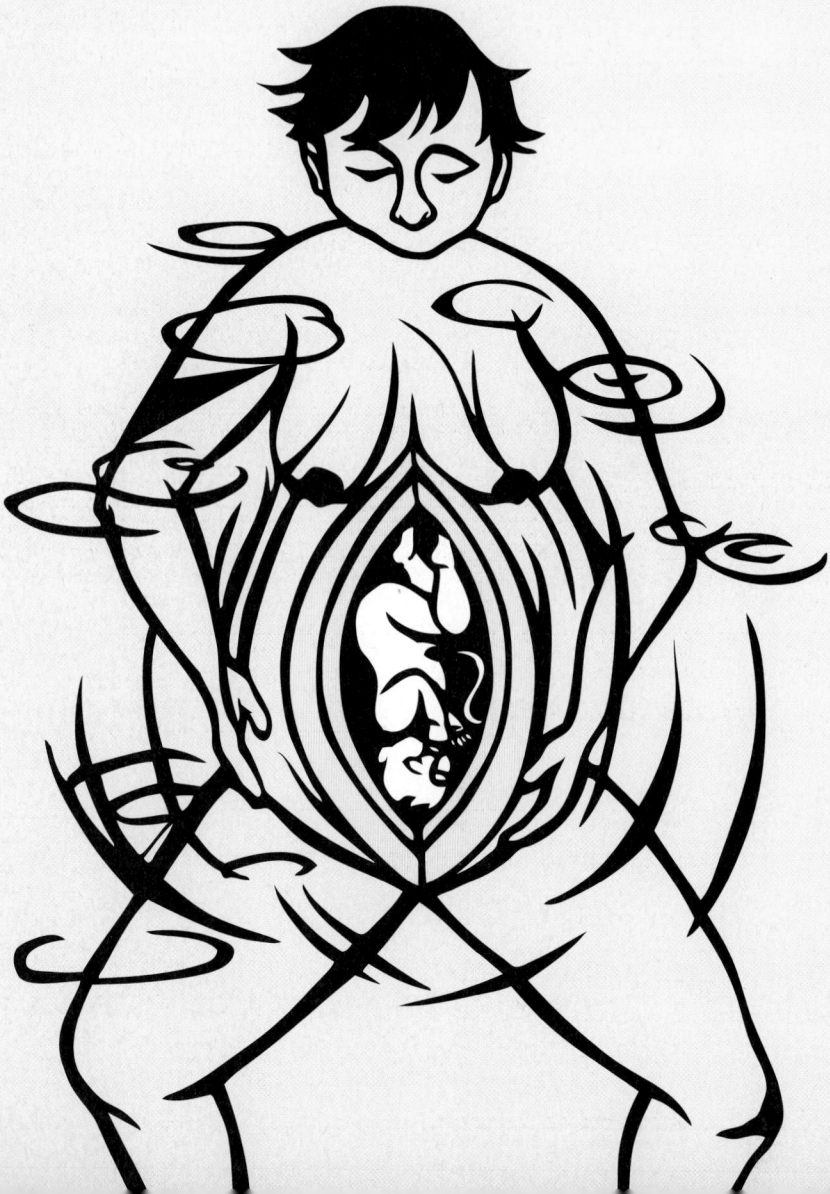

10th MONTH

my birthing story

my baby!

I am a Mother.

surrender

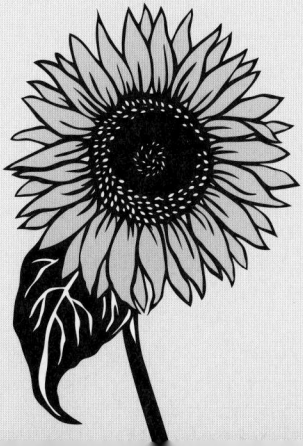

nursing and nuzzling

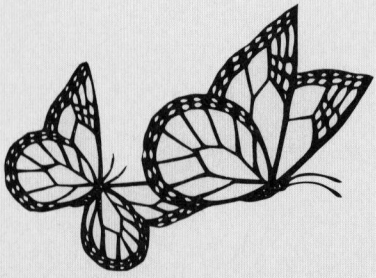

sweet baby smells and sounds

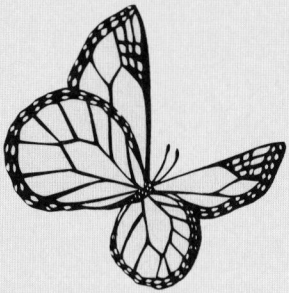

first yawn, first nap, first sight of each other

the excitement and peace of our new family

settling in

first visitors

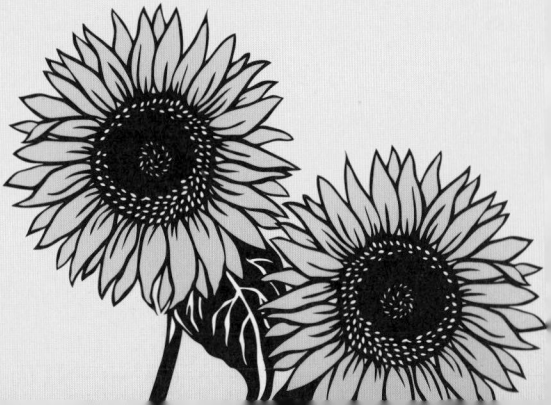

welcomes from far away

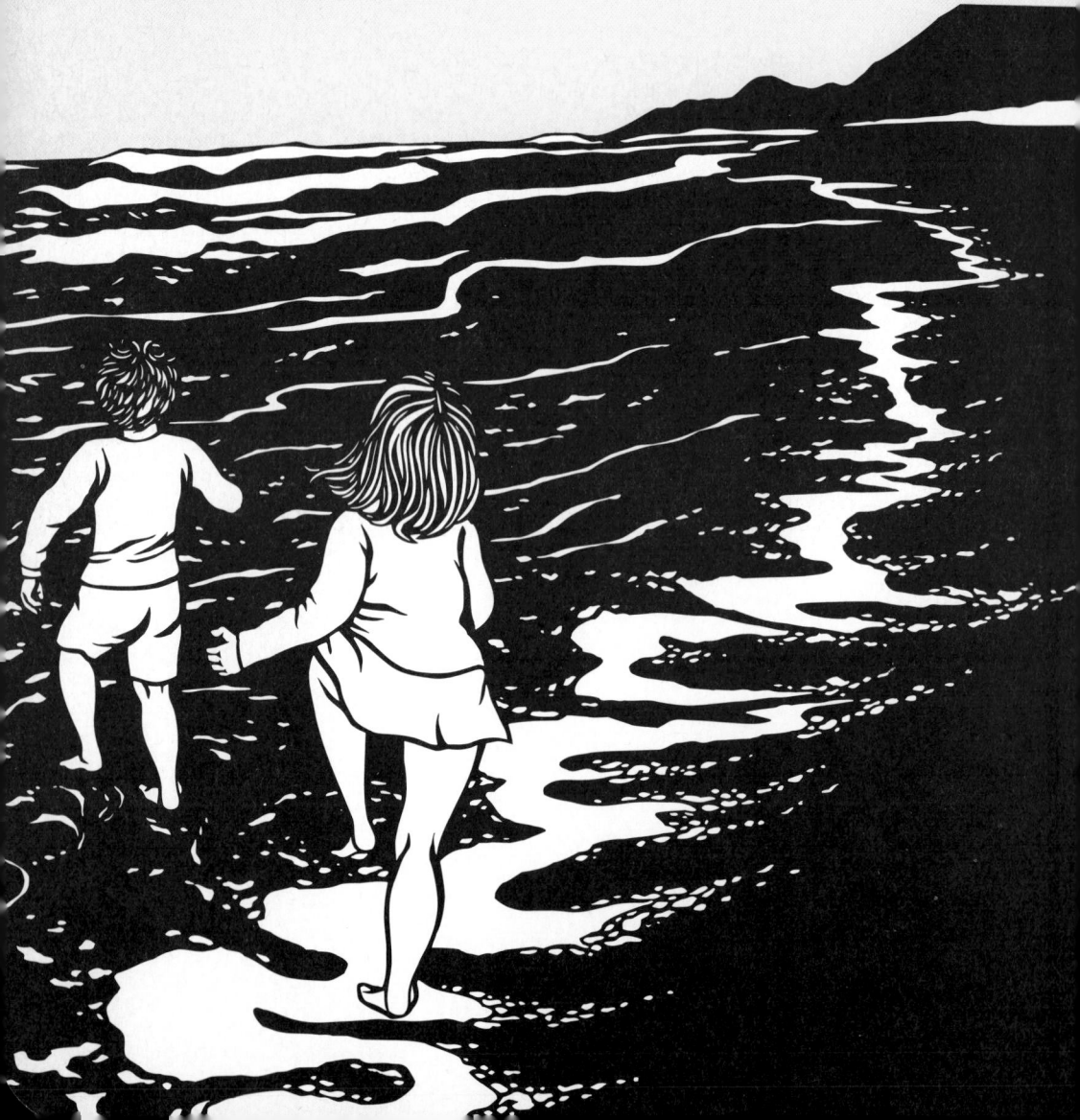

DREAMS

dreams of the baby

dreams of change

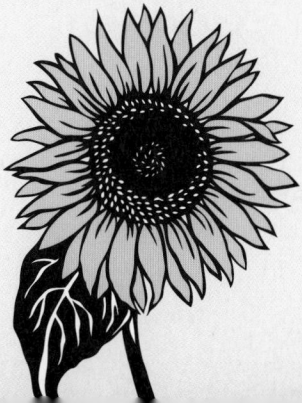

dreams of courage and trust

wishes for my child

wishes for the birth

hopes for me as a mother

hopes for my family

PREPARE

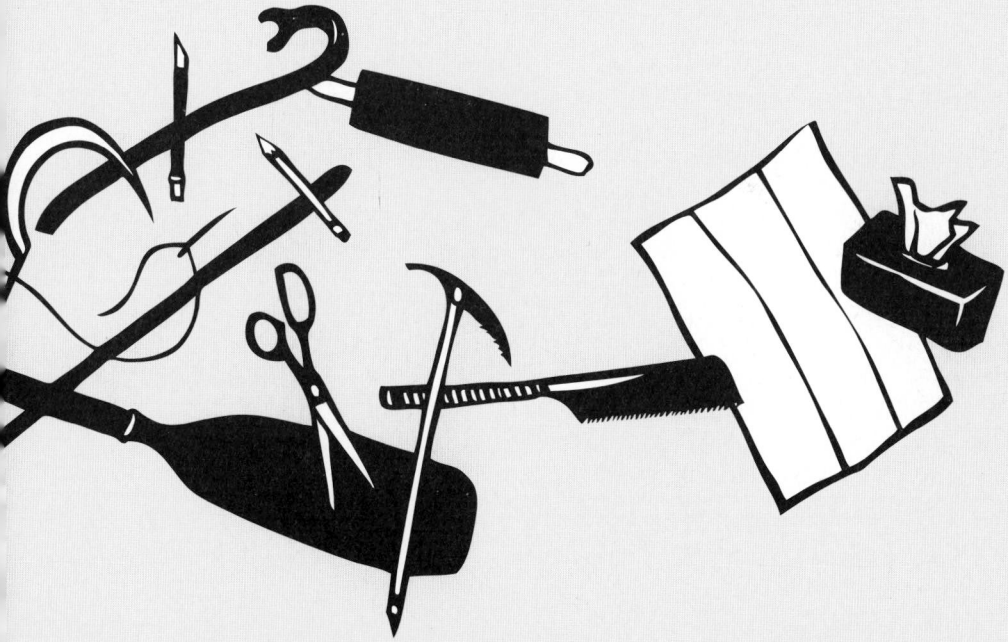

birthing supply list

all you really need are diapers
and a changing pad

Homemade Wipe Recipe

1½ cups water

1 tablespoon almond or jojoba oil

1 tablespoon baby soap (like Dr. Bronner's mild)

1 to 2 drops tea tree oil

Mix everything in large bucket with secure lid.

Cut paper towel roll in half along the middle with a sharp, non-serrated knife, removing the cardboard tube from center. Stand one half of the paper towel roll in bucket with uncut side down. Let it soak for a few minutes and flip so cut side is down. Put lid on until ready to use.

When using wipes, pull from center of roll. If you are going away for a few days, place wipes in fridge so they don't get moldy. You can also add a few drops of essential oils if you wish.

Fill a small zip-top baggie for the diaper bag. Easy!

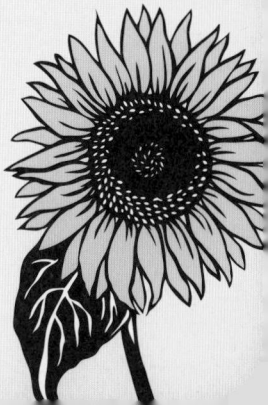

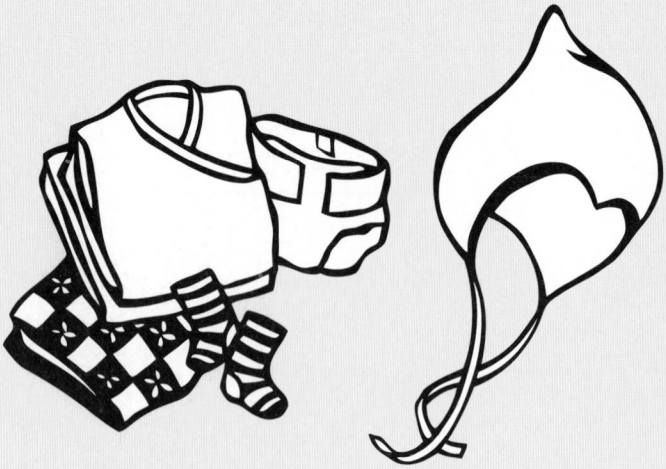

hand-me-down histories

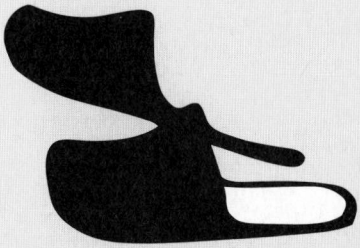

HOSPITAL BAG

robe, slippers, snacks, camera, music

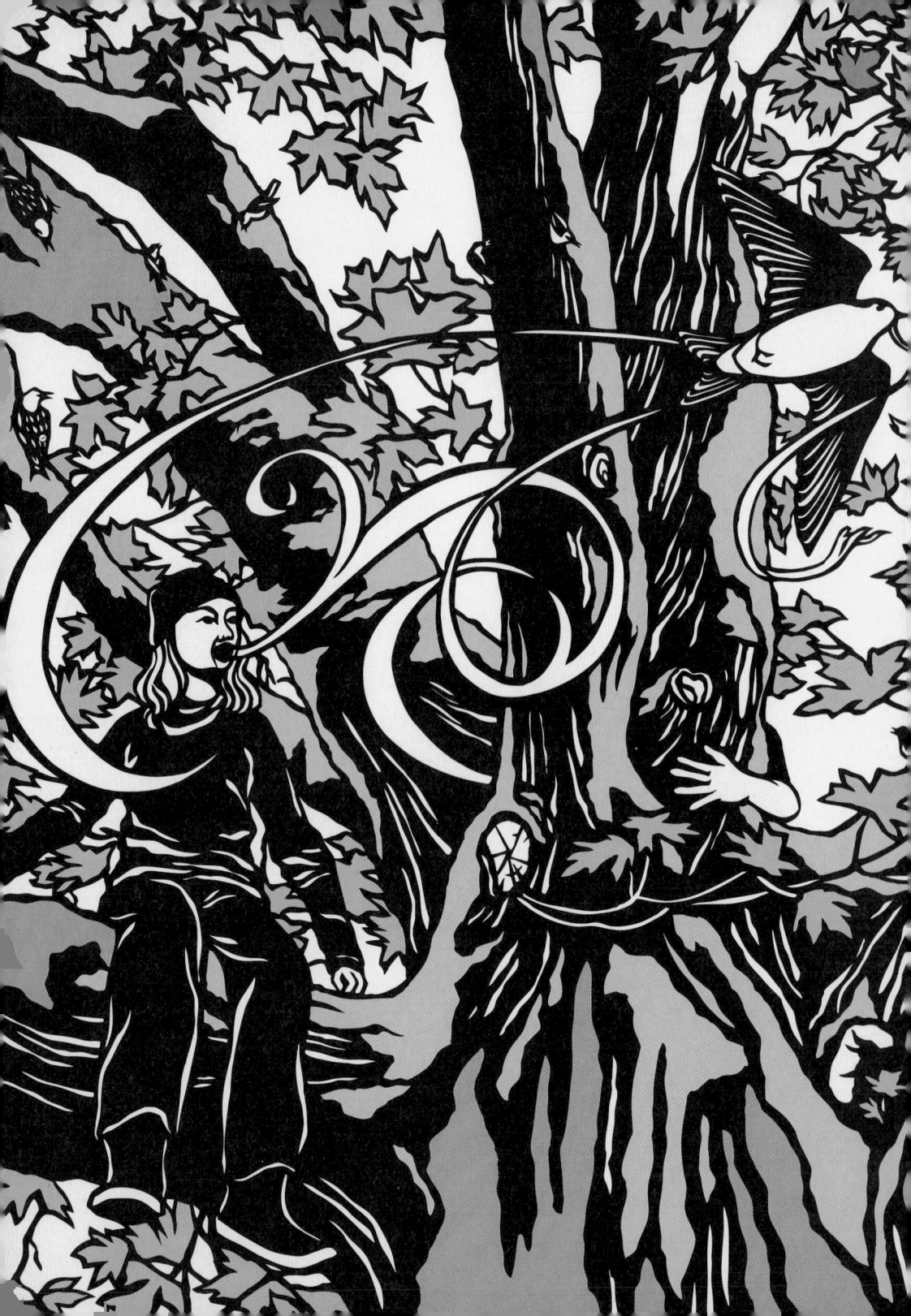

Who will spread the news?

Who wants to make us dinner?

yoga moves and stretching

crazy nesting plans

make baby's bookshelf

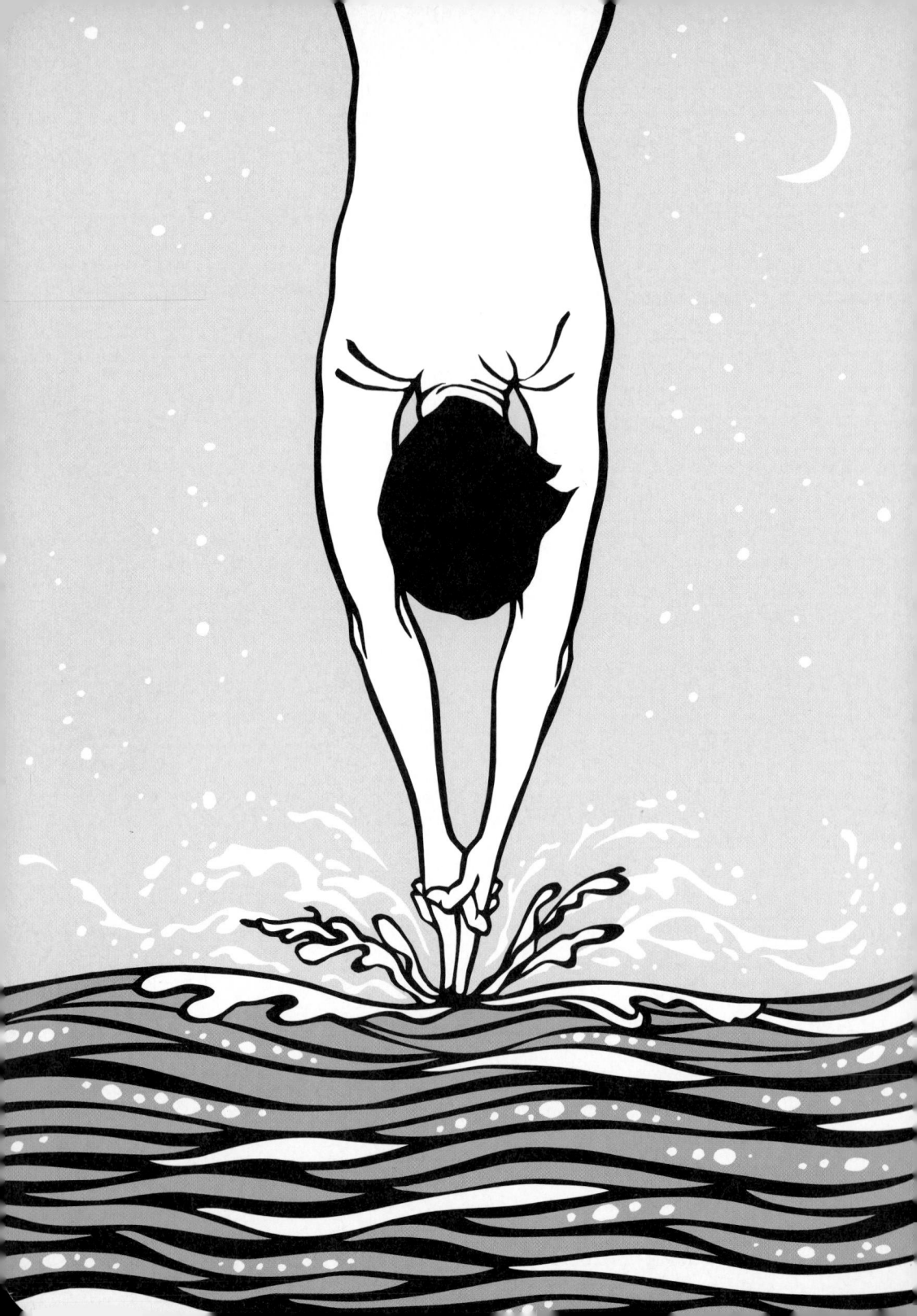

TRANSFORM

photos and drawings of my changing body

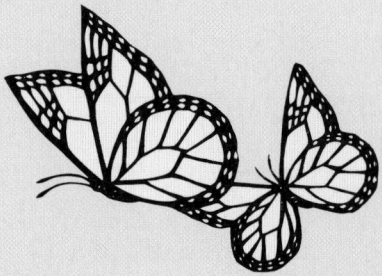

emotional changes

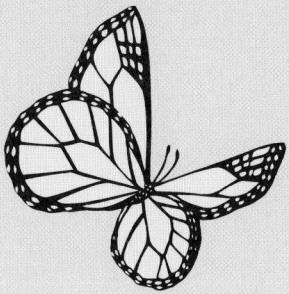

gathering courage

classes to take

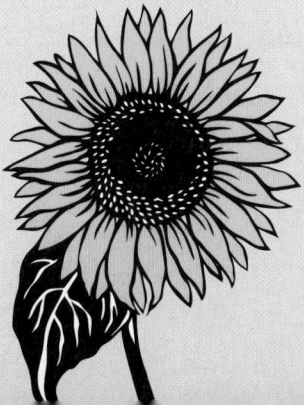

books to read

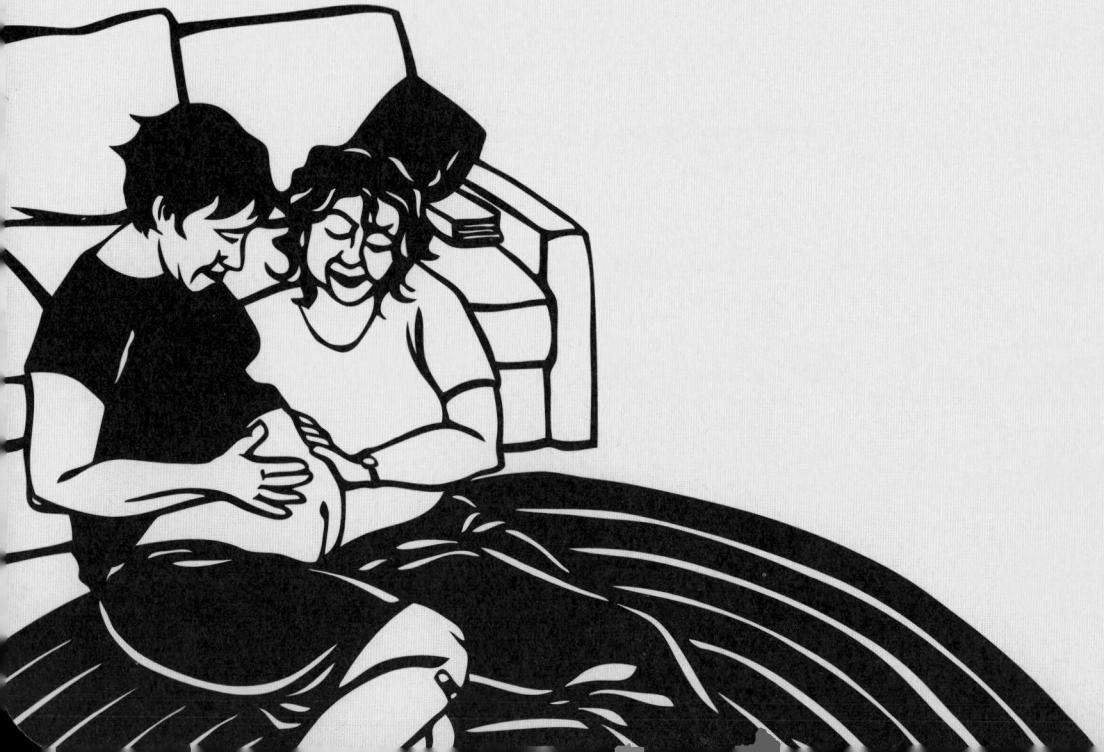

WELCOME

wishes of love for me and my baby

wishes from mothers

wishes from fathers

sisters

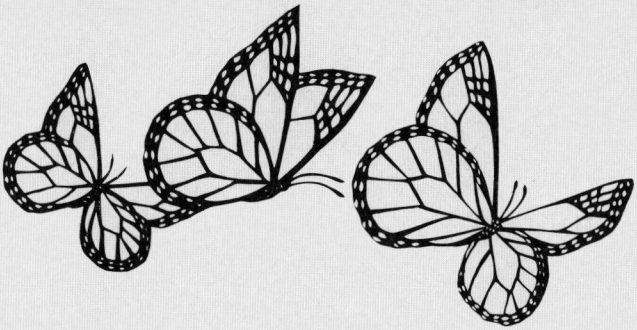

brothers

friends

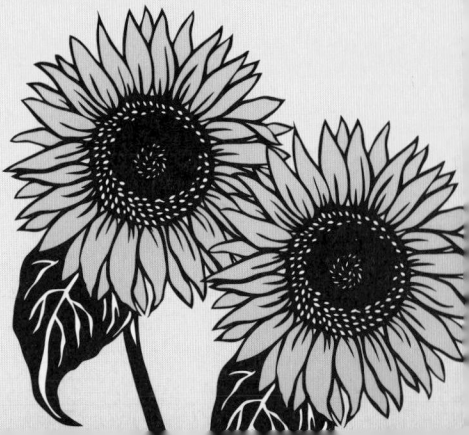

children

the whole town

score cookies from the café

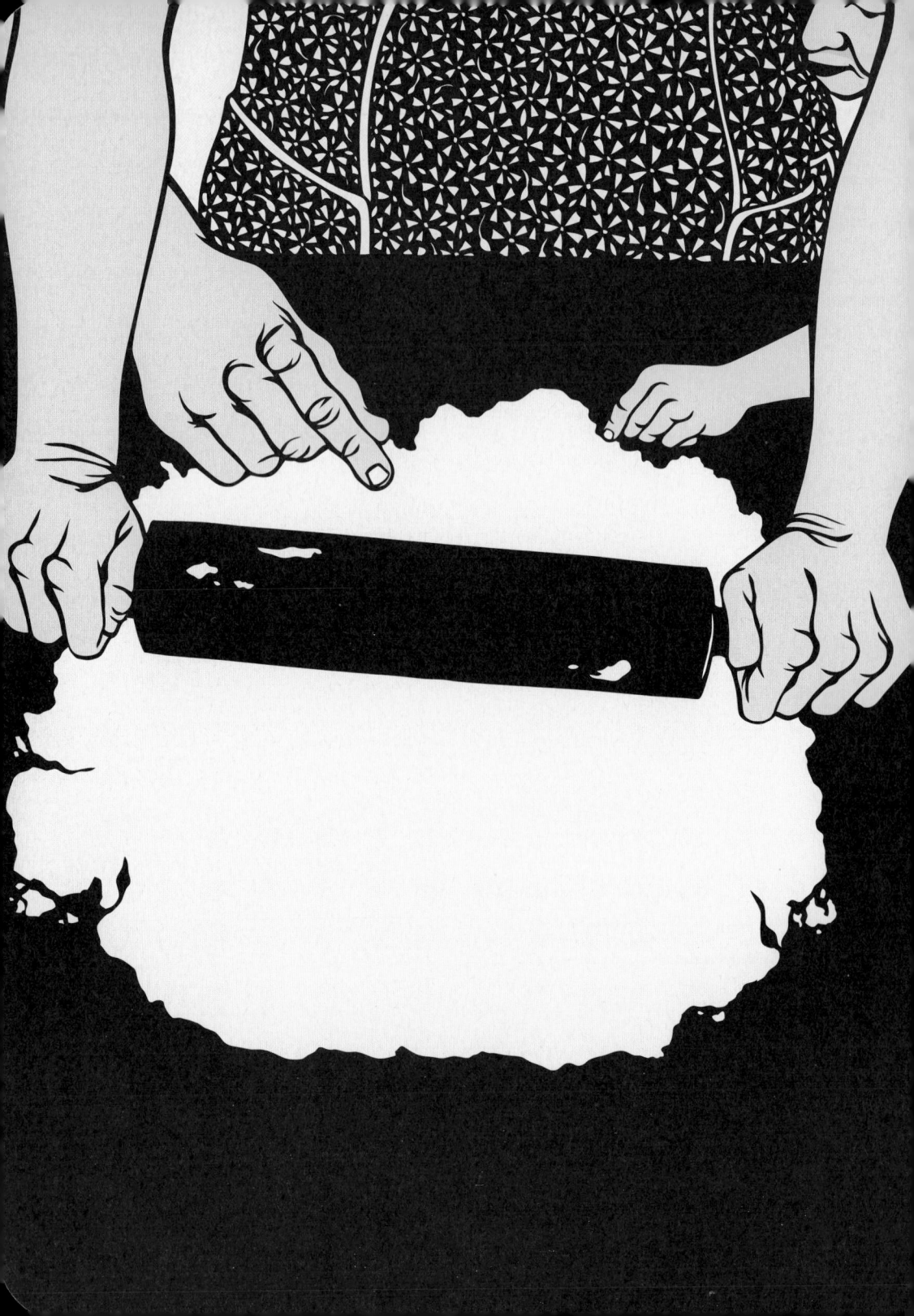

NURTURE

how I take care of myself and my baby

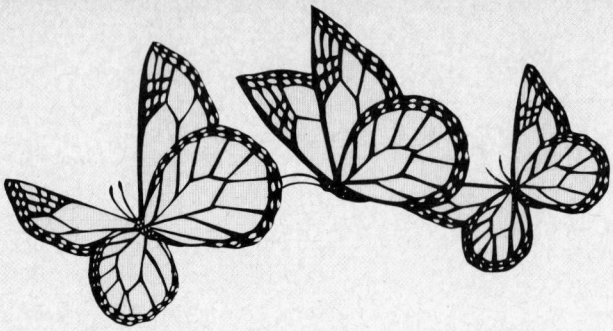

Who takes care of me?

Who takes care of my family?

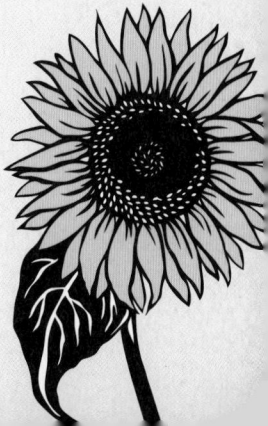

offers of help

Love. Love. Love.

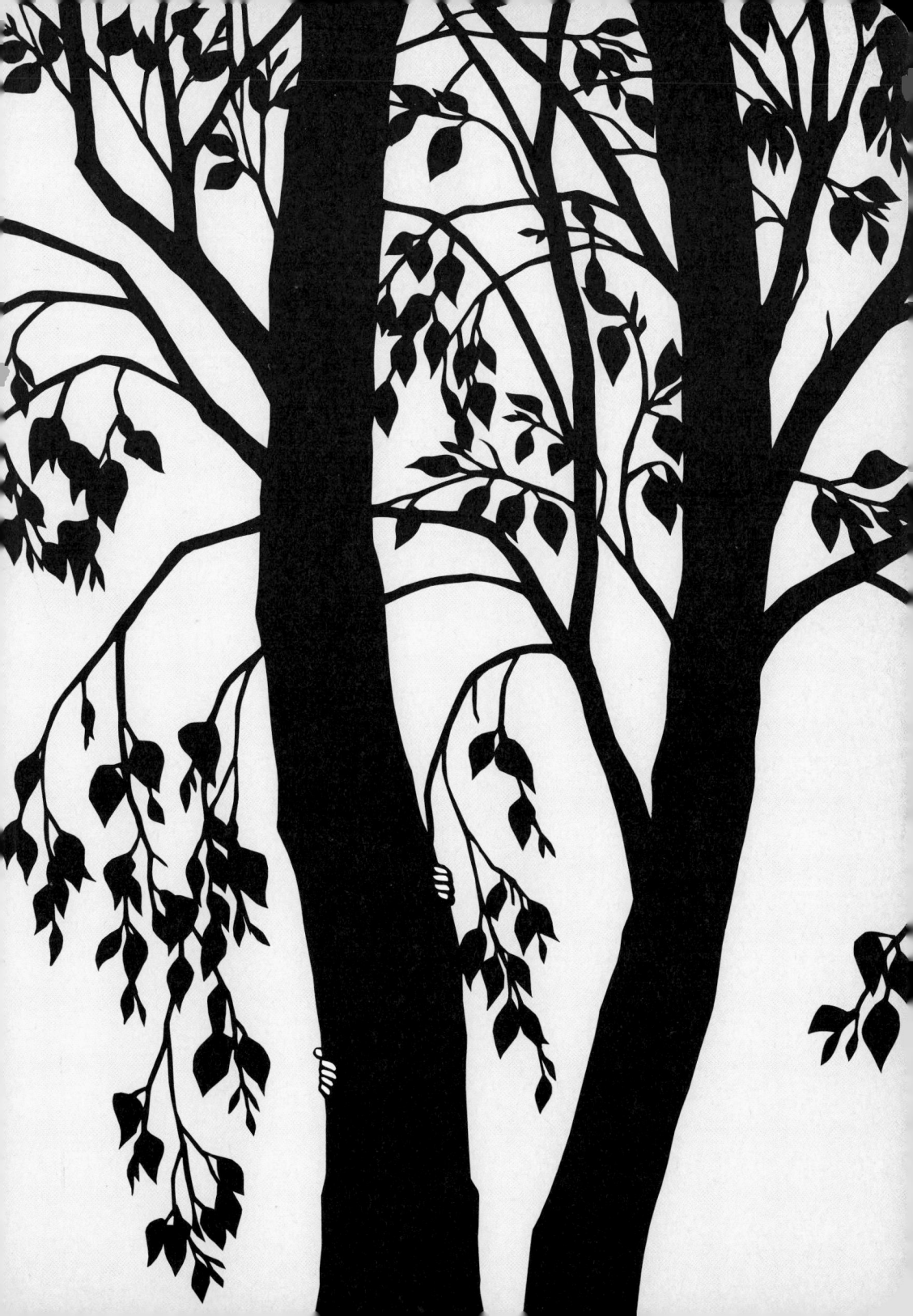

NAMES

old family names

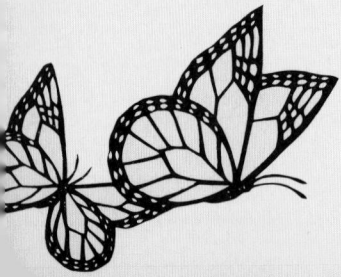

Not these ones!

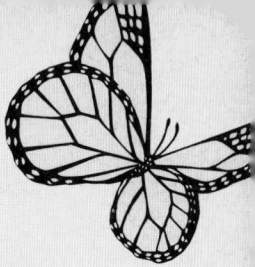

APPOINTMENTS

doctor, midwife

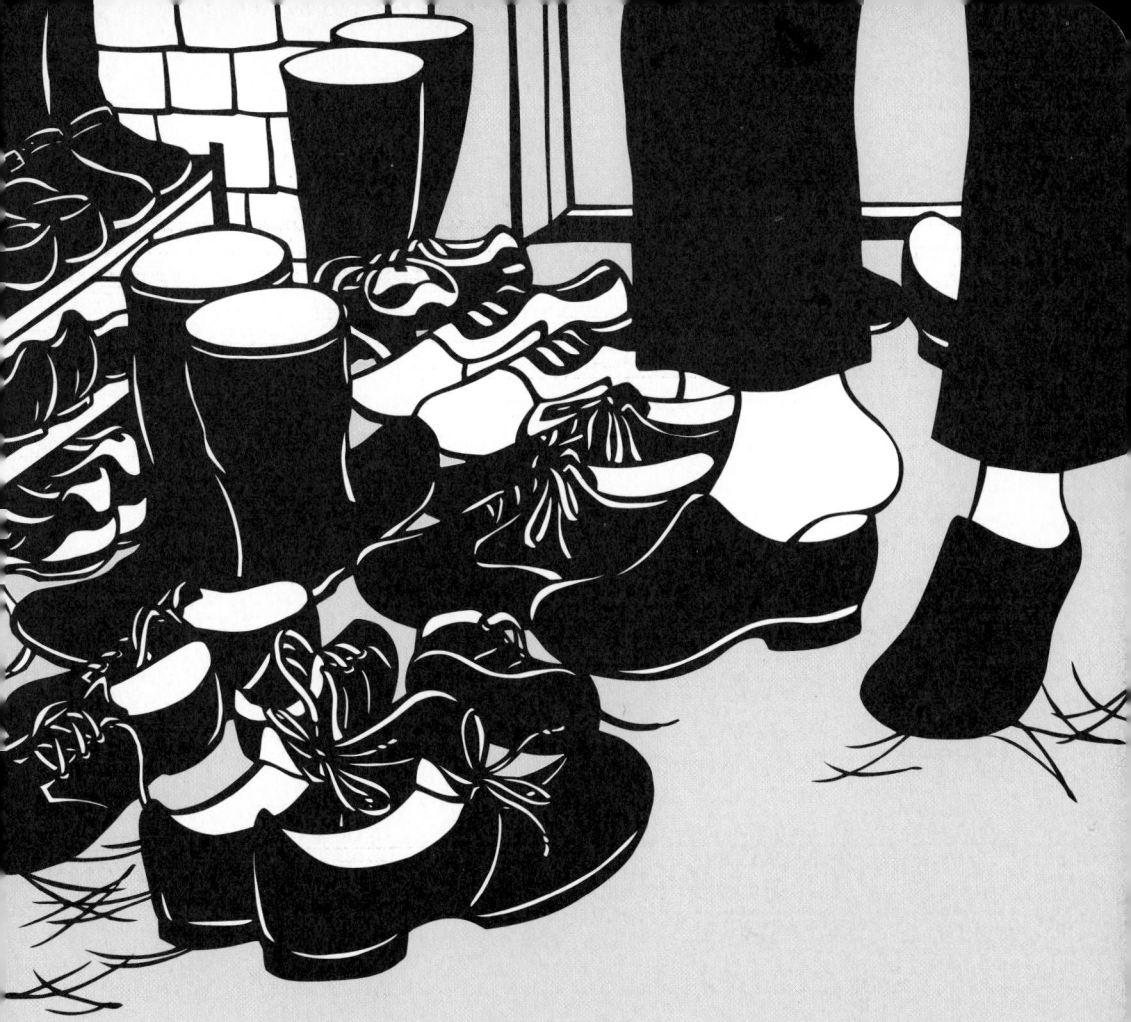

massage, ultrasound

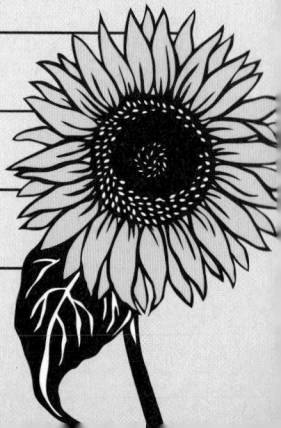

last day of work!

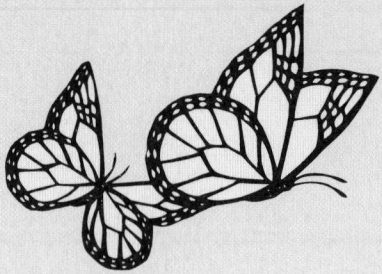

go on one last date

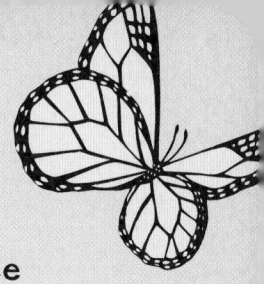

RESOURCES IN MY COMMUNITY

people and places to turn to for assistance

HELPERS

Who can I call on for help?

cleaning

making food

grocery shopping

breast-feeding

a hug when I am overwhelmed